A Poignant, Practical and Humorous Trip Through My Colon

IT'S HALF PAST MIDNIGHT

ROBERT E. CULL

ISBN: 1-4196-6452-2
ISBN-13: 978-1419664526

Visit www.booksurge.com to order additional copies.

TABLE OF CONTENTS

PREFACE

This email to my friends in the Aldersgate Sunday School Class was written in July, 2007, immediately following one of my visits to MD Anderson. As is nearly always the case, I was struck by something rather profound and moving while I was there. It serves as the most recent example of how we can choose to be inspired or saddened . . . how we can find strength and courage or choose fear and foreboding. I hope to remain open to the more constructive and hopeful messages that enter my awareness when surrounded by fellow cancer survivors.

Son, Show Me The Way

Many of you are aware that I made my semi-annual pilgrimage to MD Anderson this week. While I look forward to the day they tell me never to come back, there is a part of these visits that I will miss. They provide fertile ground for introspection and inspiration. They are full of abundant opportunities to reinforce and replenish the gratefulness I feel every day for more reasons than I can enumerate.

You have probably figured out by now that I am an addicted and unabashed observer of what goes on around me during these visits. I can't help it. I am at once both saddened and amazed by what I see and hear. The full range of emotions from laughter to choking back tears can occur multiple times in multiple locations during the few hours I am there. It will vary as to whether I will carry the image that caused me to cry or the one that caused me to smile as I think back about who I saw and what I heard. Sometimes I carry both. There are many patients and loved ones who carry books, newspapers and laptops to kill the time sitting in waiting rooms. The MDA trains run pretty much on time, but there are always gaps in the schedule. I don't carry anything because I am too busy absorbing conversations and the ebb and flow of fellow travelers along the way.

In that emotionally-rich environment, I observed a young mother and her two children. The two children, one an older boy and the other his young sister, were almost a perfect match with one of our two sets of grandchildren. The young mother looked like a soccer mom, with warmup, Nikes and hair in a pony tail. The young boy looked a bit like a modern-day Norman Rockwell painting, without the freckles. He had on a Houston Astros baseball cap sitting atop hair that obviously needed attention and a scruffy pair of non-descript tennis shoes topped by sagging socks. Little sister was much more together, from her tightly-wrapped pigtails down to her clean, pink socks and bright white tennis shoes. As I studied this threesome, with the mother reading a newspaper and the children pulling items out of a project sack, I wondered who they were here to see. Was it the husband / father who was somewhere in the bowels of MDA getting poked and prodded? Surely it wasn't the very healthy looking mother or her children. Maybe it was her father or mother . . . I wondered.

Then they called my name… "Meeestr Obur Kool"… or something like that… Asian I think. So I dutifully followed her lead to the dressing room to slip into my designer gown. After that, I took a seat in an inside waiting room until they called me into their little shop of horrors for the coup de grace of the day… a CT Scan with barium swallow and barium enema. Makes me wanta hit somebody every time I think about it. Talk about a violation of your personal space… person could get arrested for a whole lot less.

As I waited my turn, I noticed that the soccer mom and the two children had come in behind me. What happened next shocked me. The nurse came to take the little boy back to have his intravenous drip device inserted. The conversation that ensued between the mother and the nurse had to do with the fact that the little sister could not go in with the mother. There was a pause, while the mother contemplated what she should do.

The little boy, with dark brown eyes, olive skin and his dirty Houston Astros baseball cap shrugged his shoulders and said . . . "Mom, I can do it". He took the nurses hand and off they went, a kind of Mutt and Jeff look from the rear. He never blinked... he never hesitated... he never backed away even a little bit. His strides were confident and strong and more like one would expect from grownups like me and thee. Tears welled up in my eyes. I maintained my composure, but just barely.

In the ensuing conversation another patient was having with the mother, I learned that he was now 11 years old, but had been dealing with cancer since the age of seven. He had been through surgery and had been receiving intermittent radiation and chemotherapy treatments ever since. The prognosis is not good.

Sometimes we try to convince ourselves that children are naïve about such things as life and death and probabilities. While they may not be able to spell the words or know how to use them in a sentence, they do understand. This little boy, in the face of years of knowing, years of trips to the doctor and the clinic and endless focus on his disease, stood his ground that day. He stepped up with courage and conviction to go through the motions once again, and to go through them without the consolation and comfort of a loving mother nearby.

"Mom, I can do it", he said. As we individually and collectively seek the courage to go through this life, we sometimes waver ever so slightly in that endeavor. All I could think of as he walked hand-in-hand with the nurse was, "Son, show me the way".

INTRODUCTION

I am traversing a pathway littered with "firsts". It seems that everything I have experienced during my illness has been something new. It makes me feel uninformed. It makes me feel curious. It makes me angry... at myself. That last emotion comes from the fact that I essentially allowed myself to contract one of the most preventable forms of cancer (colon cancer) and turn it into a potentially life threatening situation.

The result has been a relative blur of symptoms, analytical procedures, lab work and surgery... and that was only the beginning. Following that I have run the gamut of high-tech and low-tech testing, scanning and incessant poking and probing. So far, I have survived. But there must be at least 100 trees that were sacrificed just for me to feed the paper monster we call healthcare. I have resorted to agreeing to sign the "Privacy Statement" receipt only if they promise not to give it to me.

But I feel restless. I feel that there are things I would like to say about this journey to others who are navigating the same maze, having the same feelings and trying to maintain optimism and hope in the face of this scary disease. The journey includes cancer patients, family caregivers, friends and loved ones.

My initial reaction to this urge was to scoff at the idea that I would have anything worthwhile to say about this circumstance. I am not a doctor or a clinician of any kind. I have had the good fortune to be extremely healthy throughout 66 years of life with little more than an occasional cold and a hemorrhoid or two. I had never worn a hospital gown until my colonoscopy. While the details may vary, we all share a lack of knowledge about dealing with cancer.

After giving myself permission to undertake this book, I contemplated its content. It occurred to me that I had laughed a lot along the way. There were numerous times during this process when I found myself chuckling about something (often my own condition). Thus, my belief in a couple of things: 1) The human condition is often humorous and light-hearted even in the most serious circumstances; and, 2) Laughter is undeniably one of the most effective emotions to relieve tension and move our spirits to a better place. While I have absolutely no way to prove that this is helpful in any way, one would be wasting time to try to convince me otherwise. Of course, there are times when it is difficult to muster even a smirk, much less a smile. I tried to share some of the more sobering thoughts as well.

While much of what you read here will, indeed, be my story, one lesson learned is that no one is where I am. No one carries the developmental, psychological and spiritual profile (some would say baggage) that I carry. No one has lived the same life experience I have had. And, quite frankly, most of the cancer patients to whom I have been exposed face a future significantly less certain than my own. I am one of the lucky ones who can still see a lot of light at the end of the treatment tunnel.

As a result, I tend to shy away from the "Seven Steps to Health and Happiness" or the "10 Steps Needed for Cancer Coping". I hope to be sharing, not directing. As you read, I hope that discernment travels from your inside out, not from my outside in. I hope you discover small "nuggets" that might lighten your load or create "ah-ha's" that resonate with your situation.

As we move through this material, there will be a number of places where "I Digress… ". These interludes are my way of sharing my experience and some of my communications to friends and family about my journey. Often there is humor involved. Almost as often, there is a serious note embedded that reveals those moments of doubt and dismay or fear and sadness.

The end result of my effort is a blended series of chapters that I hope will help you or a loved one negotiate these difficult circumstances. I begin this work on a serious note in Chapter I. I hope to have captured the shared emotional reaction we all must feel when we first learn that we have cancer. One of the final chapters is a letter to my children and their families as part of my Father's Day 2004 gift to them. Hopefully, in the middle you will find practical, inspirational and humorous balance in a time when the scales of life seem tipped against you.

Chapter 1

It's Half Past Midnight

It's half past midnight, barely entering February 11, 2004. It happens about this same time every night. Since I'm a night owl, it's not unusual for me to be sitting in the semi-darkness, watching a late movie I've seen before, or some thoughtless sitcom. All of this is preliminary to hitting a relaxed state that leads to a good night's sleep.

But tonight is different. I can't tell you what I'm watching, but I'm not asleep. My mind has drifted to some other place. It's a place I've never been… a place with issues and questions about life and living that I've never had to contemplate. Intellectually, I know why my mind is in that place, even though I continue to resist the reality that drove me there.

I allow flashes of the truth, interspersed with disbelief, to skip across my mind. I cling to the idea that there must be some mistake or some other truth. Those flashes are almost a blur of a mysterious symptom followed by tests and procedures that resulted in a diagnosis of… cancer… colon cancer!

That's what the doctor said. His diagnosis was followed quickly with instructions on what we would need to do in preparation for the next steps. Surgery. Recovery. Probable chemotherapy. A future filled with years of checking and double-checking my condition as a cancer patient.

"A cancer patient," I thought… "I've never even been a patient". That is true. Beyond a very rare cold or some minor physical inconvenience, I had never spent the night in a hospital room, nor had I been the object of even the most minor procedure to remove anything I inherited at birth.

I looked around the darkened room. "I am awake", I thought, followed by "this is not a dream".

Earlier that day I saw pictures of the tumor that triggered blood loss sufficient to create anemia for the first time in my life. That was the mysterious symptom that drove me to have my first colonoscopy, probably ten years late. The tumor was large enough to require surgery, but there was no way to tell, except with surgery and biopsy, whether other organs or lymph nodes were involved.

Surgery! Three to five days in the hospital! Six months to a year to get fully recovered! And then… and then… I didn't want to think about it. The light in the room flickered with the changing scenes on the television screen. I tried to watch the unknown show, but I could not focus.

Memories of my mother came rushing back. She had succumbed to metastasized colon cancer 15 years before. My grandfather was a leukemia victim. A member of my extended family died a couple of years ago from a virulent form of cancer. There are others… friends, colleagues and acquaintances… some surviving, some not… who have had their lives altered by this disease.

Now, after all these years with the constitution of a lion, I have met the equalizer. Cancer is a fearful enemy. I don't know about the statistics, but in my experience it seems to take more lives than it spares. Often, those lives that are spared have been altered by procedures and chemicals to such an extent that quality of life becomes an ongoing issue.

The light in the room flickered again. I briefly discarded my thoughts and looked at the TV screen. Again, I saw nothing.

A rush of questions filled my mind. What would I tell the family? Friends? How would I react to their expressions of worry and concern? Would I be brave? Would I show courage and fearlessness in the face of this threat? Would I cry? Heaven forbid that a tough old bird like me would ever shed a tear… even on his own behalf.

I had always thought of myself as a relatively brave person, taking on life as it comes with a fair amount of determination, grit, optimism and an absence of immobilizing fear. But, looking back, I realized that most of my life had been spent in arenas either alone or with manageable foes or circumstances. Now I am not only joined in the arena, but with a foe that is more fearful and deadly than any I have ever faced. Suddenly, life's transient and mostly insignificant crises pale by comparison. I had no framework… no context… no experience on which to rely.

I knew I had to do something. I had no idea what that meant. But I knew I would have to find out in the morning.

Chapter 2

The "We" in "I"

The good news is that when morning came, I was not alone. Rather, I was joined by my wife of over 38 years. Fortunately, Janie had many years of valuable experience working in the healthcare industry, including some high-level projects as a consultant to major hospitals. She knew the system. She knew how to make the wheels turn and which buttons to push. She could separate the players from the pretenders.

Those things represent her knowledge, gained through years of experience in the field. But the crucial attributes that would drive my treatment process would be her personal commitment, perseverance and indefatigable search for not just the right answers, but the best answers.

Many (maybe most) of us are caught flat-footed when confronted with major healthcare decisions that go beyond the routine general practitioner stage. It demands a lot of us and our partners when we are given a short fuse between diagnosis and the need for invasive treatment or a complex treatment regimen. I cannot emphasize strongly enough the need for a partner to help run interference as you try to make the best possible healthcare decisions while under the cloud of recent bad news. I simply do not know what I would have done without Janie to "block and tackle" her way (our way) through a rapid series of decisions that led to excellent treatment virtually every step of the way. Certainly, we collaborated and discussed the options, but it made my job a lot easier to have to consider only a few choices after many others had been visited and discarded in advance.

The red light indicating that our telephone was in use was lit almost continuously over the few days following the diagnosis. Friends, acquaintances, loved ones and neighbors were queried about their own experiences or those with whom they had come in contact. A myriad of questions was asked about providers, facilities, programs, clinical trials or any other subject that might be helpful in making our treatment decisions going forward. Physician and facility names and references were gathered quickly and efficiently.

During these early stages, I basically stayed out of the way while Janie pushed the decision process to the first critical level. At that point, we had to collaborate on how we would narrow the list, first for colon resection surgery and then for ongoing management of the disease to include chemotherapy and monitoring going forward. This task was made somewhat easier by the fact that she had already winnowed the list to some of the more obvious choices that combined both quality of care and convenience.

The fact that we have outstanding medical facilities and physicians near our home provided an easy transition to the first step of surgery. Janie had diligently prepared a short list of surgeons with excellent reputations and a long history of performing procedures similar to my own. Identifying the surgeon and scheduling the procedure, I found, was the easy part.

The days following were a virtual blur of activity as I was scanned, x-rayed, poked and prodded for lab tests numerous times leading to my date with the surgeon. The "busyness" did not allow much time to ponder my fate. However, there were moments along the way that were much like that first night. While I would move back and forth between optimism and serious concern, my wife would provide the ballast necessary to offset those swings. She would occasionally have to tamp down an optimistic surge to force some reality into the situation. At other times she would have to pump up a somewhat deflated spirit contemplating an altered life at best and the end of life at worst.

It is testimony to her sense of me that she was able to tell roughly when those moments were present and how much inflation or deflation was required to moderate the mood swings.

Her guidance and research did not stop with the surgery, however. We had decisions to make in terms of the extended care that comes with being a cancer patient, not to mention finding a convenient location where the near-certain chemotherapy could be administered. Again, we were served by her knowledge and the good fortune to be located less than four hours from a world-class cancer center at the University of Texas MD Anderson Cancer Center in Houston. This description rolls off the page fairly easily, but there is a maze of administrative details that must be first understood, and then mastered, if one is to gain admission to one of the foremost cancer treatment centers in the world. She did that. And she did it almost singlehandedly. My contribution was to discuss options that were virtually already resolved and then follow orders. It turned out that I was better than expected at following orders, primarily because I had absolutely no idea what to do next.

The "We" in "I" has grown to include providers, fellow cancer patients and others whose lives have touched mine along the way. It includes family and friends who offered thoughts, prayers, cards and support. A situation like this brings us face to face with the goodness of the human spirit. It reminds us that there is a magnificent world outside ourselves that provides the energy and focus necessary to overcome. "We" will, indeed, overcome.

Let me end with one final note. Certainly the path you will follow in dealing with your particular circumstance will be unique. Having said that, however, one suggestion is that the threat of cancer is far greater than any discomfort you might feel about abandoning your own personal providers or local healthcare system. Finally, remember that it is your body, your life and your loved ones that matter... not the personal or institutional ego that you will hire and pay to provide services.

Chapter 3

Other Four-Letter Words for "Ouch"

There are any number of things I learned while going through a relative blur of discovery, diagnosis and treatment in the early going. First on the list for a colon cancer patient after finding a tumor too large to suck through a straw is "slicing and dicing" (aka surgery). Janie quickly sorted through local institutions and colon "cutters" to come up with a short list.

As it turned out, the first physician on our list made us feel so comfortable that we stopped the search immediately and scheduled a colon resection procedure only a few days later. Since there were a number of tests, labs and scans required ahead of the surgery, we spent those few days going from one place to another getting my interior analyzed to a "fare-thee-well". Since there was fasting involved for a couple of days before and several days after surgery, they almost lost me to starvation instead of cancer. I knew there was some reason why I had been carrying around those surplus pounds all these years... you can never tell when you may need them.

Looking back on it, I realize that it was truly a blessing to rush the process and create so many tasks leading to surgery that I simply had no time to dwell on what evil awaited me in that operating room (O.R.). It truly seemed like one day they discovered colon cancer and the next day they were wheeling me into the sanitary confines of bright lights and blue booties. Thank God for those folks in the O.R. who dress funny. They can tolerate laying somebody open and handling all the squiggly, squishy stuff in there. If the world had depended on me for such advances, we would still have a life expectancy of 47.

My recommendation to anyone going through this process is to act quickly and overload the calendar with tasks and tests. Hopefully, this will create a blur that obscures the disquieting reality that they are already sharpening their scalpels and getting ready to put your name under the "In Use" sign on the operating room door.

I Digress . . .

This is the first of a series of emails I sent to good friends in my Aldersgate Sunday School class and elsewhere, along with family members. I hope it provides both insight and levity...

"In addition to providing some serious life experience, it is both touching and humbling to receive emails, cards, calls and other expressions of support and prayerful intervention from so many people. It is clear that we are bound together by our shared human experience, even if our paths have rarely crossed. I will be better for having learned that important lesson.

At the age of 66, it is amazing that every single thing that has now occurred is a first in my life! I had never spent the night in a hospital... never wore a hospital gown... first endoscopy, colonoscopy, surgery, morphine, sponge bath, massaging hose, etc. etc. It's a hard way to learn new lessons, but the alternative is not very attractive. I don't want to bore you with details (as he prepares to bore you with details) but here are some highlights:

In the recovery room following a serious attack on my body, the poor nurse was desperately trying to moderate my pain:

Nurse: "Describe your pain on a scale of 1-10. "
Yours truly: "Expletive, expletive, expletive."
Nurse: "I know it hurts, can you give me a number?"
Yours truly: "Expletive, 12, expletive, I have never had

> *pain this bad and can't find the words (or the numbers) to describe it. . . "*

I really can't account for (or be held responsible for) anything else that might have been uttered during those frantic moments immediately following surgery, but it could not have been a pretty picture. Fortunately they got things simmered down and gave me control over this little pain pump magic button that I could push at will (actually it only allowed doses every six minutes) to get me through the first couple of days.

I have always been a somewhat private person. However, I discovered that with disease, drugs and severe pain, one can shed any modicum of pride or privacy. Everything yields to the moment and to the task at hand. I did my daily walks down the hall with my back door open (a la Jack Nicholson)... and wearing hose, for Pete's sake!! Fortunately the wonderful technicians would catch up with me before I paraded by the nurse's station to arrange my designer gown a bit more modestly for the tour.

Thanks to a great medical and hospital team at Baylor Medical Center in Dallas, I came home on Day Five. I was surrounded by family and friends throughout the hard parts. My room was full of cards and messages from so many of you. All of these things bolstered my spirit and my will to move forward. With Janie's great help, we are doing just that. We have a few more things to deal with downstream. But the good news is that the cancerous polyp and a couple of problematic lymph nodes (out of 11) are now in a Mason jar somewhere in the recesses of Baylor Medical Center. Since I donated any body parts left on the table, some future med students will no doubt be peeking inside that Mason jar from time to time. I am glad to contribute to the field of medicine but would prefer that future donations be in cash or traveler's cheques.

I appreciate all of you... keep on truckin'... Bob Cull..."

Chapter 4

Pre and Post-Op Stress-Almighty! Syndrome

I came through the surgery in a breakeven position. I was minus 8-10 inches of colon and plus 8-10 inches of scar tissue. But nobody could convince me that those diabolical O.R. folks were not the meanest bunch in the building. The very idea that they could gang up on me (while sound asleep no less) and do stuff that created such pain and agony supports my position. Never mind that they were saving my life... IT HURT!!! Of course, you must remember that I was one of those folks who never had anything more invasive than penetrating a cuticle. I was still in possession of everything that was in my physical inventory at birth, so there was no frame of reference for this level of discomfort.

During the pre-surgery and recovery process, I learned a number of important lessons:

1. When they call your name in the surgical waiting area, play like you are someone else. Maybe you can start looking around the room as if trying to help identify the next candidate. You might even want to use one of those stick-on name badges with "Cecil Furbish" written on it (or if your name is Cecil Furbish you can use "Bob Cull"). Unfortunately, I

had family and friends with me. They immediately started pointing and calling out to the wolf in nurse's clothing that I was, indeed, present.

2. I usually appreciate preferential treatment. However, in this case, they let me know that I had been moved up because of a cancellation. Nobody explained, but I just knew it was probably because they lost the last guy in the first ten minutes and the lead surgeon simply turned and hollered, "NEXT!".

3. Don't let that scheming anesthesiologist sweet talk you into thinking it's all gonna be OK even though the early start will prevent him from making you "happy" before being wheeled into the O.R. I went in there wide awake. It all looked very clean… and verrrry stark. Thank goodness I only had time for a couple of one-liners before the lights went out. It's a little like leaving a game early with your favorite football team in the lead… if the outcome changes you don't want to be there to see it.

4. John Wayne's pain management program is (to be kind and G-rated) a load of horse manure. You may

recall that our cowboy heroes, after having been shot seventeen times, would simply take a shot of whiskey and bite down on a bullet while the good doctor removed all seventeen bullets with a rusty knife and pair of kitchen tongs.

5. Don't be a "manly-man" hero. Not only does it make the recovery infinitely more painful and uncomfortable, it may even slow the process in some unknown ways. I started out using the Wayne method absent both the whiskey and the bullet. It finally dawned on me that they gave me control over that little button for a reason. Once I became convinced that no one would think less of my manliness (took about 24 hours), I started pushing that little button with regularity. "Plop, plop, fizz, fizz… oh what a relief it is…".

6. Don't let anybody lie to you about the quality of hospital food. My surgeon was almost apologetic on about Day 3 when he approved solid food in my diet. By that time I had been fasting for about 4-5 days. My best recollection is that the menu was something like pheasant under glass, lobster,

biscuits and gravy, eggs Benedict and cinnamon rolls dripping with frosting. I may be off just a bit, but it absolutely tasted like that. I don't recall food ever tasting quite that good.

7. During the recovery period, I was periodically scheduled for x-rays or scans or lab work of one kind or another. The nice folks in the "transportation" department would show up to move me to a gurney and haul me to my next appointment. After the first trip took a while, I made a special request for the gurney driver who had the NASCAR labels on his shirt. I made several "gurney-journeys" during my stay. Our "drivers" would parallel park in the hallways outside the appropriate lab and then leave. So it was up to me to continue calling attention to the fact that I was next following the gurney just ahead. The busy attendants' smile probably hid her secret desire to give my gurney a push just hard enough to land somewhere out of sight.

8. Finally, I was not idle during all those hours of incarcer… uh, recovering from my surgical experience. In fact, I utilized my very best creative

juices to come up with a new discharge policy for hospitals. Once you're in there, it becomes clear that every patient is living for "Discharge Day". If you have never received sample medications before, you may not understand this new discharge policy. It's very simple. I suggest that every morning at 8 a.m., all patients not tethered to their room in some way all show up in the lobby. Each one will be issued a sample packet with one pill. Any patient with the strength to open the packet and release the pill will be discharged. All others will be sent back to their room. I figure if you're strong enough to open one of those hermetically-sealed little packages, you're strong enough to go home. You could probably even mow the lawn.

If I could offer a serious thought about all this, it would be that you should never be bashful or reserved about asking a question of the physician or the staff. A question for the doctors may have to wait for morning or evening rounds. But questions that can be handled by nursing staff should never require more than a half-hour or so to get an answer. It is also very helpful to have a friend or family member in the room when the physician visits since you will have been busy pushing that little button and may not have all your faculties functioning properly.

If you have had a good deal more experience than I, you may already know all this. But I can assure you that we "first-timers" have a lot to learn about managing our hospital stay.

I Digress...

An email to friends went something like this:

> *"As in every situation, I have learned some important lessons in all this. Probably the one that is most humbling and touching is the outpouring of cards, emails, telephone calls, flowers, thoughts and prayers that have come from more people than I would have imagined. Many are old and dear friends. Others have been around for some time and still others are relatively new. Surprisingly, some are even strangers who are fellow travelers dealing with similar health issues. This latter group, in particular, is full of valuable information, guidance and experience to help us make the very best strategic choices going forward. I will be contemplating this outpouring for meaning and purpose*

relating to our shared human existence. But I already know it will reinforce my sometimes vague notion of the inherent goodness of people."

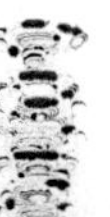

Chapter 5

A Tree Hugger's Nightmare

Years and years ago… like decades… I was a budding new sales manager with Xerox. Our professional lives depended on paper, but there was already talk of a "paperless" society, where everything would be captured and stored electronically. Yeah… right.

During this personal journey, I have experienced the fact that much of it is still talk, while some of it has actually evolved and become real. But the truth is that healthcare and its aftermath (insurance) may be more deeply committed to murdering trees now than at any point in our history. The ubiquitous "Privacy Statement", mandated by federal law, shows up almost every time you enter a different door. Never mind that you are in the same hallway in the same institution. You are presented with another copy and a request that you acknowledge its receipt. You may remember that my response was that I would sign the receipt only if they would promise not to make me take the document.

The other half of "ubiquitous" has to be the admission forms they stick under your nose on a "handy-dandy" clipboard with a cheap pen. You begin to wonder what they did with the prior 96 versions you have filled out in the last three days. You ask for, but you will not receive an admissions form "waiver". You will fill in all the blanks... every time... over and over and over... and you will enjoy it!

One of my lessons learned was to develop a very detailed, one-page cheat sheet with insurance group numbers, medications and dosages, dates and names and places for any health issue during my lifetime. That not only relieved me of having to memorize everything, it also provided my wife all the details if I didn't feel like filling in the blanks... again.

Regardless of the nature of your health insurance coverage, there is a relative tsunami of paper hiding behind "Door Number 3" just waiting for you to be dismissed. There must be some little paper cut-out guy who waits until you have left the parking garage before pulling the plug on this mountain of gibberish called explanation of benefits, statements, and so forth. It often comes in batches from different institutions, providers and payors. So far, I have received about six inches worth weighing in at something like 4-5 pounds.

I wish I had something brilliant to say about how I handled all this. The truth is that I don't speak "insurance" and operate most of the time in a complete fog as to who owes what to whom and when they are going to repossess the grandchildren if it is not paid.

I might just offer a couple of ideas. One is that you should have one place where every single financial document related to your illness is kept. Another is that I would arrange those documents by the Date(s) of Service specified as much as possible, rather than chronologically by the date received. That way, if you have to follow a particular trail for a particular service, it may be easier than hunting through a chronological file.

The final thought is that I went into this thing thinking I was dealing with one physician and one institution. That was true. What I did not account for was the 427 (or was it 428?) different radiologists, labs, consultants and others who participated in the tiniest slice of my healthcare pie. I only began to get nervous when Vito's Pizzeria, Top Hat Dry Cleaners and the Cloud 9 Massage Parlor showed up. I'm kidding, but the truth is that I have had a hard time figuring out exactly what in the world some of these folks had to do with anything. Good luck with that!

Chapter 6

And for Our Next Act . . .

If you are paying attention, it is no doubt apparent to you that I am the "dufus" of healthcare. That dubious distinction takes a lot of conscious effort... don't think about it... don't ask about it... and, most of all, don't listen to anyone in a position to know better. The result is that I actually thought the invasion of my body and subsequent removal of the "bad guy" (along with 8 inches of the "good guy") meant that I could go home and never go back. Surprise! Shortly after surgery, our first visit to the center of excellence resulted in a prescription for 12 bi-weekly chemotherapy sessions. They wanted to assassinate any "critters" lurking in places undetected by the battery of tests and exams they had administered.

***I Digress** . . .*

Another of my emails to friends and family:

> *"First let me say that I continue to be grateful for your thoughtful and prayerful expressions of support as we continue to turn over every rock on our way to what we hope will be a successful conclusion.*
>
> *We spent three days this week at MD Anderson. My sense is that they have a "test inventory" list somewhere and they*

simply start with the "A's" and stop at the "Z's". They poked and probed and photographed my insides and outsides, and drained and measured fluids of every kind emanating from every orifice in my body. If there was any material that did not emanate on its own, they would simply drill a hole and suck it out. In every case, they were the "pokers" and I was the "pokee". I was also the "probee" and the "drillee" and the "scanee". After three days, I just automatically took off my clothes when entering the clinic and looked for a line in which to stand (a little overstated, but not much).

The good news is that the data collection phase is pretty much over. The neutral news is that we will not find out until Monday exactly what this all means in terms of next steps. We know chemo of some kind will begin very soon, but not sure if a bit more surgery will be required on a second site until we get the biopsy results. Janie is doing a wonderful job of pulling together a range of choices relative to oncologists and programs available in the Dallas/Fort Worth area that will maximize the effect of the MD Anderson findings and treatment recommendations. It is wonderful to live in an area where our biggest problem is narrowing the list to one out of many excellent individuals and programs.

Before I go on, I would also like to say that I do not know what I would have done without Janie. She is knowledgeable. She is thorough and aggressive in her search for answers. She is the best advocate anyone could ever have to help move through a difficult and sometimes scary process. It is largely due to her efforts that we have moved along this challenging path with both quickness and quality. I appreciate her loving and caring (sometimes requiring a stern countenance dealing with both patient and providers) attitude and commitment. I am more convinced than ever that she is testimony to my good taste.

Finally, I must address the card (an original with art work by a class member). Let me say that I believe there may be a case here for invasion of privacy. Otherwise, how could anyone know that I had a heart tattooed on my tokus (that's Okie for tush). Further, I do not comprehend how anyone who has seen my stunning physique could ever depict me as some ordinary, somewhat overweight and rather squatty specimen of a male child. And, last but not least, I intend to enlist Mack (an attorney and class member) to determine if there is cause for an artistic malpractice suit. Outside of that, I thought it was cute... OK I thought it was <u>r-e-a-l</u> cute... OOOKKKKK I even laughed out loud... With love and appreciation... Bob."

As you could ascertain from the previous email, our "center of excellence" is MD Anderson Cancer Center, part of the University of Texas system in Houston, Texas. We are so fortunate to have a world-class institution so close to our home, and will be forever grateful for that access. As I discussed earlier, our plan was to establish a baseline view of my condition following surgery (x-rays, labs, CT scans and the like) with MDA and continue to return for those tests and future colonoscopies. Given this association, it seemed natural to utilize a sister organization (UT Southwestern Medical Center) in Dallas to oversee and administer my chemotherapy regimen.

***I Digress** . . .*

With test results in and a new phase beginning, I just had to share with friends and family once again:

> *"As you know, we went to Houston again Monday, 3/29, to hear the news coming out of our week of medical gymnastics. Right off the top, the great news is that the second site is benign. There is a name for it (a gang of something or other). The important thing is not what it is, but what it is not.*

Once Janie and I stopped doing back flips and high fives (and I put my clothes back on after learning that there were no tests on the schedule), we discussed the future of our treatment regimen and also came to a decision about ongoing care. In addition to sharing the UT designation in both Dallas (Southwestern) and Houston, our physician is acquainted with a leading oncologist on the staff at Southwestern. We will meet with him Monday and will likely start chemotherapy either that day or very soon thereafter. We will know more after our meeting as to the frequency and length of treatment that will be required to maximize the result.

Speaking of results, what we are really talking about are probabilities. I don't know about you, but I was in a constant state of "yawn" as my statistics instructors did their best to penetrate the fog. We are all vaguely aware that life expectancy continues to evolve as we reach certain ages, but most of us don't give it a lot of thought. Until, that is, we are confronted with the big "C". All of a sudden, we become extremely sensitive to the connection between various treatment strategies and the effects of each on the probability that we will be around in three years, five years and beyond. The truth is that 20 years ago I would have wagered against my being alive at this age. Now, however, I am offended by the idea that I may not live forever. Funny how expectations change and how we dig in our heels a bit when we begin to realize that red sign at the end of the tunnel reads "Exit".

But my hope is to follow Wayne Dyer's advice. That is, "... don't depart this life with your music still in you." Well, I have been a bit preoccupied in recent weeks, but I hope to extract a symphony before moving on... or maybe at least a jazz band... ukulele?

Thanks to each of you for the cards and thoughts and prayers that keep coming our way. I cannot tell you how touching and encouraging it is to Janie and me as we go forward. It is a constant reminder of your caring and it propels us forward with the energy and commitment required to maximize those probabilities... with appreciation... Bob."

Chapter 7

Chemicals I Can't Spell

I Digress Already…

At the outset of chemotherapy, I informed some close friends:

> *"We met with the oncologist yesterday at UT Southwestern Medical Center in Dallas. I am scheduled to get my infusion port installed tomorrow morning and will get my first chemo treatment next Monday. As I understand it at this point, I will spend one day every other week for six months (12 sessions) at the facility and will carry a pump for 46 hours after each session. Given the chemical cocktail I am taking, this should give me about a 70-75% chance of non-recurrence at three years. If I hit that mark successfully, the percentages go even higher, until at five years they figure I'll have to get run over by a train… or at least something other than this colon cancer will have to cancel my ticket."*

A portion of the first day of chemotherapy is spent in orientation with one of the experienced nurses who will be administering your chemicals. I am sure they assume the patient has a healthcare IQ of something brighter than a 40-watt bulb. Thus I am also certain they were privately discouraged with yours truly. I couldn't pronounce most of the chemicals (save magnesium and calcium), certainly couldn't spell them (oxy something, louca something) and was embarrassed each time I repeated the other one (5FU). To this day, I don't know the right chemical name for that one. I just claim I can't remember in order to avoid a startled response like "same to you, buster", or "6FU to you!".

Seriously, this initial visit is where I made one of my many mistakes along the way. The nurse told me everything I needed to know but her knowledge exceeded my ability to understand and retain all of it. As a result, I was many weeks into the treatment plan before I began to get the full picture of what they were doing and what I could expect as a result. Let me recommend that you don't succumb to the feeling that you can just go along for the ride. Stop the discussion as many times as necessary to ask for clarification, take copious notes and don't leave there without a very clear picture of the treatment and its potential ramifications.

I Digress...

I related part of the orientation to friends and family in the following excerpt:

"Now for today's lesson... 'necessity is the mother of invention'. We all know that one. Well, at my first session, the nurse was trying to educate me on the vagaries of chemotherapy and what I could expect during the process. After she explained the pump part, she said I would be bathing in the tub on the two days it was hooked up. I softly but firmly explained to her that I had not taken a "tub bath" since something called a bassinet. I honestly believe that I started taking showers when my little legs would hold me up long enough for a wash and rinse cycle. And I never bought into the program that one could get clean while wallowing around in his own dirty bathwater. Bathtubs are for loungers, and I'm not a lounger. My specific intent while growing up was to wash off today's dirt, watch it disappear down the shower drain and get my body ready for the next sweaty, dirty little game day... soooo, I found another use for sandwich bags and duct tape.

I simply attach the tape to the plastic bag, leaving enough sticky surface around the edges to stick to my skin and then press the duct tape firmly in place. I have pulled out most of the chest hairs in that area. So I suffer little at this point when ripping off my Rube Goldberg sandwich bag and tape device. It's a little tricky to leave the pump outside the shower and stretch the tube to its limit while I'm on the inside, but I'll do almost anything to avoid wallowing in that dirty water. So, contrary to the UTSW party line on pump carriage and bathing, I want all to know that I have not wallowed around even once... now, if there are no further questions... Your Friend Bob."

One of the important reasons why chemotherapy "first-timers" must get a grip on any likely side effect is that some of this stuff is powerful and can yank your physical and mental self all over the family room. It's one thing to deal with something you know is "normal" or somewhat predictable as a side effect. It's a good deal more unsettling to experience a side effect without that understanding. Do your homework. Ask a lot of questions. Take a lot of notes. Raise your healthcare IQ to that of a flood light.

Chapter 8

Ports and Pumps

One of the steps that had to be taken prior to chemotherapy treatments was to install a port through which they could feed all the chemicals intravenously without having to punch a new hole in my veins each time. While I resisted the idea of another incision, it became clear over time why this "docking station" was so necessary for intensive chemotherapy. Inserted just under the skin, the nurse could simply plug into it and then hook and unhook the various bags of "goodies" with very little effort. It was relatively painless going in and coming out and the lump was located just under the strap on my tank top when cavorting on the beach... yeah... right.

I Digress...

An early update for friends and family early in the chemotherapy process went as follows:

> *"I'm one day past my second chemo series. Every other week this consists of one day in Dallas - about five hours - and two days with a pump at home. The first series was almost unnoticeable. I snorted and roared, beat my chest and talked loud on the telephone. 'What side effects?', I wondered aloud with a sneer and a snicker.*

Today. . . well today I feel a bit like a furball in the middle of the living room floor. . . already composed of undesirable elements and only awaiting some kind of harsh cleansing chemical to sweep me away. I promise to be more respectful of the 'side-effected' among you who have traveled this road before me. I will talk softer and make note that my body is not impervious to being hammered with the 'heebie-jeebies' or the 'botz'. I will also (and this is a biggie) cease pointing my finger and giggling at those blue-haired folk who discuss their. . . uh. . . oh, well. . . bowels. . . all the time. I have discovered there are moments when it is difficult to think about almost anything else.

I wasn't going to share any other stories with you today, but remembered one experience on my way to chemotherapy.

Some of you may know that I had what's called a 'port' installed that serves as kind of a permanent 'docking station' for the intravenous treatments. It keeps them from having to use veins over and over and is very useful for treatment over time. Almost all of you know that my lifelong inexperience with health issues and procedures makes me blissfully ignorant of virtually every known disease and medical procedure.

The port is installed under the skin and positioned properly to deliver chemicals into the bloodstream. They (promises, promises) said I would be awake - but happy - throughout the procedure (sure). I woke up with the doc and others milling around my cubicle. Once they were satisfied that I was alert and ready to go, they left the room while I dressed.

Side Note: The port was placed near my shoulder on the upper left. Because of the location, they allowed me to retain my Speedos (kidding… just the regulars) under my designer gown. I was one happy and comfortable camper. The thought occurred to me that I had evolved from being embarrassed to take off my shirt in front of strangers to being comfortable in my underwear. Next thing you know I'll be performing at Chippendale's… give me a fire pole and a strobe light and who knows what might happen.

I dressed and returned home. As I was changing clothes later, I noticed a chrome-plated sort of nipple thing (like the male part of a snap) protruding from under my left arm toward the back. It was surrounded by a strong adhesive tape. I touched it but had no idea what it was. Several hours later I found another in about the same location on my right side. After a nap I found a third a bit lower on the right. Janie was at work so I had no one who could take a closer look.

I had visions of the mad doctors installing a port and then running all manner of tubing through my body to pop out in various locations. I had obviously not understood something about this port, this procedure and how this thing was going to work. Concerned, I called both a friend and the oncologist's nurse to describe in some detail what I had discovered post-installation. My friend had no idea but made me promise to call back once I figured it out. The nurse was greatly puzzled until, at the last moment, she laughed out loud. Then she patiently explained that the surgical team had simply failed to remove some of the taped-on connections for the EKG that were in place during the procedure.

She was stifling a laugh and apologized, saying that she was not laughing 'at' me. I told her she might as well because I certainly was. I thought it was hysterical and shared the story several times. I thought you might enjoy it, but I am confident you will not be as derisive as some of my close family members. I am expecting a higher standard of behavior from Aldersgate members and would not expect to hear words like 'idiot', 'dufus', 'moron' or 'IQ challenged' coming from that esteemed group.

It is helpful to have friends who are willing to listen while I do something that literally helps me feel better physically. Thanks for listening and I'll see you all soon. . . Bob."

Chapter 9

Left, Right, Left, Right

It has taken me a while to realize that we are all like human snowflakes. We may be similar in some ways, but none of us a is an exact replica of any other. Certainly that applies to our physical bodies. But it also applies to the way we deal with life's "curve balls". So, while I have my way of dealing with stuff, there is no assurance that any of that will be helpful to someone else.

The title of this chapter captures one of my basic tenets in dealing with virtually any crisis known to man. When I was younger, I had this terrible habit of looking at the end of things and then becoming discouraged when measuring the distance from where I stood to that end. I finally learned that successful end games are comprised of many interim steps taken one at a time. Thus my strategy in dealing with chemotherapy and the calendar is to keep my head down and never stop moving physically or mentally.

There were any number of ups and downs during the process, but the discipline of the calendar and the tasks to be completed helped me to work through this process with the illusion that time was actually accelerating. I will talk later about how I play "mind games" with myself and "self-talk" my way to a faster conclusion, but for now…

I Digress…

At some point along the way, I became aware that they were putting a jigger of steroids in my cocktail as part of the regimen to control nausea and provide a little gusto. The email to friends and family that follows let's you know that it worked:

> *"I decided that one more quick note wouldn't hurt. There is one thing that has been going on with only passing mention on my part. That is, the good doctors at SW Med School are providing me with 'legal speed' (aka steroids) every other Monday as part of my 'cocktail'. Am I writing too fast? I am so quick today, I fear that the email will show up as a blur on your screen. If it does, let me know and I'll resend with a governor to slow it up a bit.*
>
> *This stuff is GREAT!! I mean reeeeaaaallly GREAT!!!!! Just to give you some idea, here is my list of 'To-Do's' for the day:*

1. *Wash the windows*
2. *Wax the car*
3. *Clean the attic*
4. *Sweep the attic with a whisk broom to be sure to get all the cob webs, dirt etc.*
5. *Vacuum the house (floors, ceilings, walls, roof)*
6. *Clean baseboards with a tooth brush*
7. *Mow, edge, fertilize, water, aerate the lawn*
8. *Chain saw dead tree and trim all other trees and bushes in our yard and in the neighbor's yard on either side*
9. *Call Buck Showalter and let him know that I am available to pinch hit home runs on Tuesdays*
10. *Call Bill Parcells. Let him know that if they ever invent Tuesday Night Football to make me the #1 quarterback*
11. *Pick up groceries*
12. *Drop off laundry and cleaning*
13. *Call everyone in the family to wish them a "Happy Tuesday"*
14. *At precisely 4:30 p.m. crash and burn in a heap of sweat and minor delirium*
15. *Use second wind that arrives about 7 p.m. to help me stay awake half the night.*

I hope I haven't written too fast. Gotta go... gotta go... gotta go right now... things to do, places to go and people to see... So Long (zooooooooom!)... Bob."

Chapter 10
Left, Right, Left, Right… Oops!

"The best laid plans... often go awry". That is true even when one has his head down and is methodically going through the motions to what we hope will be a successful conclusion. One day a shot rang out. The shot came during a conversation when I had just finished a fine verbal exposition concerning the medical merits of my condition and the prognosis for the future. I had included all manner of conclusions about why my situation was unfolding the way it was and the precise expectations that should be part of the mix.

"You do recall that you are a Stage III cancer patient, don't you?", came the reply.

Silence. Then more silence.

Then with a bit of a "harumph" I pointed out that I was a IIIA, and that means I was just barely over the line coming out of Stage IIB. The truth is that inside I was a bit shaken by the comment that had blown my cover and shoved the circumstantial reality in my face. But this was not the first time this truth had been exposed, nor would it be the last. All the other times, the person doing the shoving was me.

I promised early on not to play the role of a victorious cancer "chest beater". While you can tell that humor has a great deal to do with how I view the world and how I deal with challenging situations, it would be disingenuous to say that I made this journey without fear or without feeling discouraged and concerned.

There were quiet moments and any number of points along the way when a feeling of unease would come over me. Sometimes the cold blade of fear would come out of nowhere, triggered by a comment or an event or a suggestion of human mortality. Just as often, it might gradually manifest itself during a quiet moment alone when my thoughts would wander outside the mental discipline of "left, right, left, right . . .".

There are numerous professionals who have a lot to say about how one should handle grief or fear or discouraging developments. I am not one of them. However, I do have some thoughts that could be helpful as you ponder your own feelings.

One of the mistakes I made in this process was that I

followed the John Wayne approach mentioned earlier in connection with physical trauma. But this time I applied it to very normal, natural emotions. As many male children are wont to do, I tended to go through my days with great bravado, spending a fair amount of my time on the banks of that river in Egypt. While I believe that denial is a useful tool to assist in maintaining a more positive and constructive focus, it cannot be the only mechanism, nor can it be impenetrable. Realistic and practical denial is to acknowledge our circumstance while pushing ourselves along a path of seeking solutions and "best practices" every step of the way. Unrealistic denial is like whistling through the cemetery... it may make you feel better but the end result is unaffected.

I Digress . . .

This just seemed like the right place for this email to friends and family:

> *"All of you know that I thoroughly enjoy preparing my little updates. I do laugh at life a lot and use humor to lighten my load. It gives me a great deal of pleasure to share with friends and family, hopefully lightening their load as well.*

But something happened that gave me pause. One of my friends outside Aldersgate responded to my last couple of notes by saying that I was 'amazing' (referring to how I was handling my health issues). For reasons that I don't fully understand, this made me uncomfortable. I don't think of myself as 'amazing'. I think of myself as a rather ordinary native Okie dealing with life as it comes and simply trying to make the best of a not-so-hot situation.

When I was at M. D. Anderson for several days, I walked the halls and ran the healthcare maze with young people, mid-lifers and old people who shared a common disease. But the variations are many as one moves from one type of cancer to another and certainly there are differences in terms of how advanced the disease has become. I literally saw people being treated who were kind of orange, flushed bright red or a frightening gray color that one associates with people who are approaching death. I saw people with no hair and so pale that they looked like ghosts. I saw people with masks covering their nose and mouth because their immune systems were so impaired they could ill-afford to breath the same air without some kind of filter. Some had loved ones with them. Others were alone.

I find the same thing as I go through bi-weekly chemotherapy visits to UT Southwestern. Some people cannot move about without a walker or some kind of support. I see the same colors and effects, only on a considerably smaller scale.

All the while, I feel good. I suffer from a couple of very minor side effects. My energy level is good, my appetite is good and my color is what it has always been. My hemoglobin has reestablished itself in the normal range and various other indicators are moving in the right direction. I walk fast into the building and walk fast out of the building five hours later. Except for the inconvenience of carrying a pump for 46 hours (until about mid-day Wednesday), I suffer very little at the moment. I am surrounded by wonderful friends and family.

My mother died of metastasized colon cancer. It finally had spread to other locations in her body, including her brain. I was not with her at the moment of death, but I was with her in the last hours as she approached the end of her life. I recall that she would sit upright suddenly from time to time and I would hold her and reassure her that I was there. I did not realize until years later (based on a similar situation in my extended family) that one of the final insults of this awful disease is that patients often lose their sight. I simply cannot even deal with how that must feel to know that you are preparing to die and suddenly you cannot even see your loved ones.

In my view, my mother, my extended family member and those fellow travelers (the red ones, the orange ones, the gray ones, those in wheel chairs, those with masks on) who are kickin' and bitin' and pushin' and shovin' and scratchin' out one more day and one more treatment praying for a miracle... they are 'amazing'. I am not. I am one of the lucky ones. It is important that you know I understand that and that I am deeply grateful to be doing as well as I am. Thanks for listening... Bob."

Chapter 11

A Side Trip

What follows gives just a brief idea of where I am in the chemotherapy process, before embarking on a rather disconnected (but I hope enjoyable) piece of attempted humor.

I Digress…

"Now that my #1 emailperson has returned from vacation, I wanted to send something along on the 'Halfway There' anniversary on Monday, 6/21, of my 12 scheduled chemo sessions. Always feels good to start down the other side and head toward zero.

Everything continues to go very well. I feel good and side-effects continue to be minimal. Of course, there are no guarantees with any of this stuff, but I am so very grateful for the fact that I have continued to be productive and have maintained normal daily activities virtually without a hitch. I know there are many whose prayers and thoughts are with me and that has to be a positive force in my journey toward a healthy future.

I also have other news. Both the Gimp (that's me) and the Gimpette (Janie broke her foot a couple of weeks before leaving for Italy) have returned from 10 exciting days of living life to the max. Janie returned this week from points that were 6-7 hours later than Central Daylight Time and several thousand miles east of Mansfield, Texas. I didn't pay real close attention, but her destinations had names like London, Milan, Florence, Rome, and Siena. She went through airports with names like Gatwick (sounds like a dry hackin' cough) and rode buses and trains (aka public transportation) and drove 'itty-bitty' rent cars with five passengers and a gross of luggage (probably looked like a Chevy Chase vacation movie). She said she didn't have a bit of trouble with the language until someone opened their mouth.

The Gimp was also pursuing exciting life alternatives during the period, culminating with a reunion with the Gimpette a half-hour late after he had waited at the wrong end of the International Terminal. After being struck with a cane, the Gimp apologized and they blissfully pecked one another on the cheek and hobbled off to the car.

It was an exciting moment, with many tales to tell. The Gimp was so excited to tell Gimpette about his trip to Dallas for chemo. There was also a quick visit to Anderson's barbecue, a day trip to Glen Rose, lunch in Granbury and a dozen other scintillating experiences (watching the rain come down every single bloomin' day in every single bloomin' way, a trip to Super Walmart to look at hardware, software and underwear, cleaning out the gutters, arranging for lawnmower repair, a visit from the pest control guy, watching The Godfather for the 926th time and the need for a new condenser... among many other spine-tinglers).

After not having taken a breath for several minutes, I finally yielded the floor for the Gimpette's recitation of her trip details. She went to a lot of places where there was a bunch of old stuff (old buildings and old art and artifacts). Janie didn't explain everything but I believe artifacts are detailed facts about the old art. They just try to make it sound fancy by putting that "i" in the middle. It sounded like most of the stuff there had its beginnings somewhere around the same time as dirt. As I understand it, the streets were narrow and traffic was heavy (sounds like NY). Everyone spoke the language (except it wasn't English until they got to the town with the airport named after a dry, hackin' cough). They didn't have barbecue over there (and very few Taco Bells or Steak and Shakes) so they had to settle for local culinary fare that was mostly Italian. In England, they must have had Long John Silver's because she made several references to fish and chips. At least they could understand each other when ordering.

When they were looking at the old buildings, she talked about some guys with names like Mike (I believe his last name came from a barbecue place in Fort Worth called Angelo's) and some other old artists like Rembrandt and others whose names are misspelled. Lots of pictures to look at, but she didn't mention any important works like 'Dogs Playing Poker' or 'Mansfield After Dark'. I'm sure the colors were nice, but how old can the stuff be if it's not in black and white?

They didn't even get to stay in hotels or condos some of the time. Nobody left the light on for them either. They had to stay in places like villas and chateaus and stuff. Instead of a highly polished professional staff catering to their every need, they had to suffer things like traditional families (even a couple of really old matriarchs) asking them what they wanted for breakfast. Had to eat outside in places like verandas (the bugs must have been terrible) overlooking grape vines and other landscaping that probably cost a fortune to water and fertilize.

For some reason, she seemed apologetic about having traveled to such wonderful world locations while I continued a routinized and rather mundane existence in Mansfield. Maybe she's right. Maybe there is something over there that goes beyond Walmart, beyond Dallas, beyond barbecue... that is more interesting and spectacular.

Now, as most of you know, I am not one to whine about very much. But she has convinced me that I may have gotten the short end of the cane on this one. So I need to enlist your participation and support. Help me begin to beat the drum right now to make me a part of the traveling party the next time there is a trip to one of those old places. It will not be easy, but I am sincere when I ask you to (I can't believe I'm going to say this)... 'win one for the Gimper'... Your friend Bob."

Chapter 12

Mind Games and Fuzzy Math

You may have already surmised that I have relied heavily on mental discipline, focus and humor to help me get through this challenge. That is one piece. The other piece is deception, deceit and distortion (3D's). We all know there is 60 seconds in a minute, 60 minutes in an hour, 24 hours… you get the drift. I have invented Situational Time Management (STM) to alter the perception of time such that benchmarks appear closer than they really are and the time required to get there seems to move faster.

I Digress …

> *"A long-time friend asked me for an update this week and it occurred to me that I hadn't sent anything along to the Sunday School class lately. The subject line gives a hint as to how I trick myself into moving time along faster in my head than it actually passes at my feet. Funny how we always complain about time passing too fast and accelerating all the time… until we are involved with something we cannot wait to get behind us. Maybe 'situational time management' would be the right term.*
>
> *With 12 sessions scheduled, I have number 5 coming up Monday, 6/7. My 'STM' says that the very next session will be the halfway mark!!! In my head, I'm already*

there... it will take a couple of weeks for CDT to deliver on that promise.

In any event, I continue to tolerate chemo pretty well. In fact, the past two-weeks (I live my life in two-week segments these days), I felt great. Truthfully, I have had very, very few days when I have not worked through my 'to-do's' and normal daily activities pickin' 'em up and layin' 'em down. I am very grateful that my side effects have been minimal.

The character of my hair seems a little different, and it appears to be thinning just a bit... but hangin' in there so far. Please understand (in deference to my 'folicley (sp?)-challenged' fellow travelers) that one can continue to be a handsome, dashing babe magnet with or without fur on top. It's just that mine has been with me this long so I would just as soon keep it... see you all soon... In friendship... Bob."

Further evidence of my ability to warp time to my own ends can be found in the following email. It also offers insight into some lessons learned along the way and philosophical eye-openers that will accrue to my benefit for the rest of my life.

I Digress . . .

"Any of you football watchers out there have seen team members holding up four fingers as they change ends before beginning the fourth and final quarter of the game. Well, I've got four in the air, since I have just completed session # 9 of the prescribed 12 session total! What I know that no one else knows is that once I have completed the one following my next session, I will only have one more to go. See how easy it is to cipher your way to the end result?

Truth is, it really feels good to see that the light at the end of the chemotherapy tunnel is coming into view (this is assuming they will draw blanks on scans and will tell me to go home and never come back). Also, I'm pretty sure that is natural light and not that of a choo-choo train (I must be spending too much time with the grandkids) heading my way. Of course, I will have to maintain regular checkups going forward. But that's a little deal.

For the moment it's just a little bit more "left, right, left, right. . . . " to the ceremonious final unhooking of the last pump three bi-Wednesdays from now (three bi-Wednesdays sounds a lot closer than six weeks). I'm thinking about buying a round of ginger ale and Snickers bars for the nursing staff and the valet parking guys to mark the occasion. But, I ain't hangin' around for fun and fellowship... I will 'high five' anybody I can reach while dashing (there I go exaggerating again) for the front door. I will be thanking everyone along the way and immediately forgetting names, locations and treatments. It's one of those deals where one is eternally grateful for wonderful, high quality healthcare institutions and caregivers but absolutely cannot wait to get the heck outta' there and pray never, ever to go there again!!

This trip has been unique and valuable in a number of ways. It finally penetrated the fog created by my thoughtless assumption of immortality. It finally occurred to me that I just might be vulnerable after living so many years as a fortunate recipient of a constitution made of steel. It made me focus much more intensely on some unfinished life business in a number of different ways. It changed my willingness to give precious time to emotions, causes and topics that should never have been very high on my life list.

Maybe most importantly, your responses, thoughts and prayers made me recall the inherent goodness of the human spirit. They have served as a reminder that friends born in the context of a search for goodness and spiritual growth are unlike friends acquired from any other environment.

There is much good to be derived from this experience and I intend to focus my attention there. I am grateful for the lessons learned. I am grateful for the prayers answered. I am grateful for the reminders of valuable life elements that had been pushed into the background. I am grateful for the timing since I can now devote all my energies to health management and recovery. I am grateful for the tremendous advances in treatments that have occurred in the few years preceding my illness. I am grateful for the minimal side effects arising out of the chemotherapy. I am grateful for family and friends who have been lovingly supportive from the outset. I am grateful that I have not been taken suddenly without the opportunity to experience these life lessons and reminders. In summary, I simply find it very difficult to complain. . . .. In friendship. . . Bob."

Chapter 13

I'm Dead and No One Knew My Feet Hurt

One might look at the chapter title and wonder why on earth I would be talking about things like death and sensitive feet at a time like this. I'm obviously not dead. If I were, sensitive feet would no longer be an issue. It is not the first time two disparate dots have connected for me in a conceptual "aha". In fact, my children bestowed the title "King of the Analogies" on me when I struggled to tie life experiences together in an attempt at effective parenting. Hopefully, we will arrive at the end of this piece with some kind of common understanding that will be useful to the reader.

If you are a cancer patient, you are acutely aware that hearing the initial diagnosis creates an aftermath of concern, fear and emotional upheaval in a variety of ways. Not the least among these emotional responses is the stark reality of one's own mortality. All of a sudden we have thoughts about being a lot closer to the end than we are to the beginning. We begin to think about all the unfinished business still on our plate. We think of all the things we intended to accomplish that now could be threatened by a debilitating journey to our final resting place.

Most of us shake ourselves free from this downward spiral when we embark on a complex, intense and serious action plan designed to get rid of the disease. As we focus on testing, procedures and treatments, we tend to push most of those negative thoughts into the background. I am convinced that is helpful and healthy, both in an emotional sense and as an aid to recovering our physical health. I do have a "however" however. Or, using the qualifying phrase of the day, I will begin my insight with "having said that".

Having said that, there is one link in the chain of emotions that we need to carry with us and act on every time we get the opportunity. It is something that most of us acknowledge as constructive and important throughout our lives. However, it is also something at which many of us fail miserably as we slide through the years dealing with the here and now of everyday life. The problem is not that we lack or deny the knowledge or awareness that physical life is not infinite. Confronted with the facts, we would all intellectually admit our mortality. But most of the time a vast majority of us keep our feet firmly planted on the banks of that river in Egypt. We figure if we don't talk about mortality, life will go on forever. It is inconvenient to contemplate the end of one's life and what that means in terms of administrative and legal housekeeping, if nothing else.

It is very important to clean up any legal or administrative clutter before it is too late. However, that task pales in comparison to the thought that there are so many important things we need to communicate to those about whom we care. Of course that would include family, but there are numerous friends and colleagues for whom we feel a particular affinity for one reason or another. A "mortality check" tends to reveal the fact that we have been mostly derelict in these particular communications, and that we could exit the planet without having said so many important things to those who will remain. Love, appreciation, forgiveness, values, encouragement and gratefulness all come to mind as elements of those messages we need to send. A critical first step is to forgive ourselves for not having done a better job while we percolated through life.

But the critical second step is to make a list of those who need to hear from us, the content of our message to them and how we will deliver that message. Some things can only be said face-to-face, either in groups or individually. Others may require a letter and still others can be accomplished with modern electronic technology (aka telephones or email). But they all require thoughtfulness, preparation and action… and action . . . and action.

So one of the dots that needs connecting specifically deals with communicating with family, friends and fellow travelers. The second dot reinforces the notion of the critical role communications plays every step of the way. Through the following illustration, I hope to convey the responsibility the patient has for clarifying health status at any point along the way.

One of the potential side effects of my particular chemotherapy is neuropathy. That is the loss of feeling in some nerve endings, particularly in the fingers and toes. This can extend to the soles of the feet as well. It can manifest itself either in numbness in those areas or in a heightened, almost painful sensitivity.

Late one evening I walked into the garage barefooted on some important mission. I stepped on a very small pebble on the garage floor and recoiled in pain over something that would hardly be noticed under most circumstances. It occurred to me that no one but me was aware of the pain I sometimes felt, even if they were generally aware of the ailment. It occurred to me that if I tried to explain it to someone, I would have difficulty choosing the words that would convey the "feel" of intense pain growing out of something so small. But, I also knew that if I wanted or needed someone to understand, it was my responsibility to find those words and communicate that understanding.

The "aha" came as I understood that I could die without anyone knowing my feet hurt... because I had not told anyone. That is the miniscule "truth". The larger, dot-connecting, screaming truth is that I could die without having told those whom I love and admire how I feel about them, about life, about our relationship and about prioritizing values.

All of that came from a small pebble and a sensitive foot. If you are a cancer patient, you need to know this. If you are not a cancer patient, you need to know this. Hmmmm... another "aha".

Chapter 14

Time Flies... I Digress

The emails I sent to friends and family during the late stages of my chemotherapy conveyed the emotion, the spirit and the lessons of this six month trek through chemotherapy. I will let them speak for themselves.

I Digress One . . .

"Yesterday I sat for the 10th time at UTSW. It was one of <u>those</u> Mondays. The Dallas traffic was unbelievable. For some reason I was not on the schedule, resulting in a two-hour delay. Traffic was again horrible on my return because the start time pushed me into evening rush hour. I waited at a railroad crossing for close to 10 minutes on the way home. You get the picture. And, of course I brought my old '46-hour friend' (the pump) home with me to wrestle with until Wednesday afternoon. On arriving home, Janie got to hear me grouse around for a few minutes about the fact that the world had been 'plum' (and I mean 'plum') ugly to me all day long. I couldn't think of another four-letter word that would be appropriate for such an august body.

And, as you might (or might not) guess, I am thrilled. I feel a bit like Lance Armstrong, peddling past #10 and headed for the finish line at #12. I figure I'm wearing the yellow jersey so long as I'm not throwin' up, livin' on the throne, vacuuming hair off my pillow case every morning or otherwise falling short of relative 'normal' every single day. I can smell it... I can feel it... almost there... almost finished. And wouldn't you know that my last session falls on a date with my lucky number... Monday, September 13!

That brings me to why I'm updating everyone. I asked some questions of the doc about next steps as we go forward from 9/13. Essentially it lays out this way: 1) I will have my first scan about 30 days or so following completion; 2) Colonoscopy on books for February; 3) Scan to be performed every six months for next five years. That is the point at which a lack of recurrence gives one a clean bill of health with normal life expectancy, but every year that passes increases probability of total recovery; 4) Will do labs and physical every three months for the first two years and every six months for the remaining three years; and, 5) the port (my old friend they installed in my upper left shoulder through which they feed my intravenous chemical cocktail) will be removed at about 90 days after 9/13. I suppose they leave it in until they have the results of the first scan and follow up physical. I have not informed the doc yet, but I will let him know soon that removal can be expected precisely on the earliest day possible. They may be planning more treatment, but I am not.

After the doctor had shared all this, he said that if I cleared all those hurdles, it would be 'bye-bye'. I told him that I really did like him, but hoped never to see him again for the rest of my life. Being the good doc that he is, doing what he does, he understood perfectly. He hopes for the same thing.

OK class, if there are no further questions... In friendship... Bob Cull."

I Digress Two . . .

"I was going to leave you alone this week. But I am so excited to be within two weeks of a complete 12 session plan that I just had to share. Almost without exception, I have dreaded my every other Monday session in Dallas and carrying the pump for another 46 hours. Maybe it was a reminder of my illness when I would prefer to believe that my feeling good meant there was absolutely nothing wrong with me. Maybe it was the inconvenient and sometimes bothersome side effects. Even though they have been few and minor, their presence probably also served as a reminder

of an uncertain future. So, while I was anxious to move ahead quickly through the process, I nevertheless felt a sense of dread in the few days just ahead of each scheduled session... until last week.

As I began to realize that there would only be one session left after 8/30 (two more measly weeks), I felt excitement and impatience as I tried to speed up the process of getting to 8/30. I could hardly wait. I didn't take a deep, sighing breath as I walked into the Center. I smiled at the valet guys and the receptionist and everyone with whom I could make eye contact. When no one was around I just looked at the floor with a little grin on my face. I couldn't wait to announce to each of the nurses that this was my next to last visit. It was truly a great day! Maybe Wednesday 9/1 will be even greater... at that point, I will only have 12 days to my last Monday session, and 14 days to the final unhooking of my friend 'Pump'!... See you soon... Bob."

I Digress Three...

"Most of us are doing all we can do to stay up with our own calendars, much less track a second one. Thus, you may or may not be aware that last Monday-Wednesday represented the final chemotherapy treatment out of 12 that

were prescribed... 24 weeks of anticipating 5-6 hours on a Monday, 46 hours worth of 'pump toting' and a return trip on Wednesday to get unhooked. It has been verrrry regular, verrry predictable and easily undertaken on a left, right, left, right kind of progressive basis. Since my side effects were not incapacitating (although I was a little more tired toward the end), it was relatively easy to keep my head down and focus on the steady counting down of my inconvenience... 12, 11, 10.... 6, 5, 4... 3, 2, 1.

As you know from a previous email, I was really pumped as I approached that final 72 hours of pouring killer chemicals into my body. It was an exciting milestone. It was the end of a series of events that started with anemia, a colonoscopy, surgery and days of diagnostics back in February and March. It was truly a wonderful feeling and I shared my excitement with anyone who would listen.

Based on my historical email pattern, one (including this 'one') would have predicted an upbeat, somewhat humorous email to hit the electronic mailbox almost immediately after the nice nurse unhooked me and saw me race (one of those relative terms) out the door. It's been a week. I know there is no obligation to report (and some of you probably wish

I would stop). The delay was caused by my inability to understand my own feelings. They were unexpected. Their character would be called subdued. Their personality would be called apprehensive. It feels strange. The counting was over (or so I thought). It was unexpectedly (on my part) anti-climactic.

I now realize that I had virtually shut the door on any cancer-related thoughts beyond those 12 sessions. It helped me stay focused on the task at hand. It helped me to stay positive as I peeled off those calendar pages on my way to September 13. But it delivered me to a place where all the thoughts, all the possibilities and all the uncertainties poured in on me virtually on the same day. It was as if I was wakened with the startling news that I had (present or past tense... I'll take the latter) cancer... cancer! I know a lot of survivors. I also have buried a number of friends and family. There is absolutely no medical reason at this time to believe that I will not be a member of the former group.

I will continue to believe that I will be walkin' and talkin' with hope and a smile until someone tells me differently. But I have to tell you that my immediate post-chemotherapy feelings surprised me and forced me to take a step back as I absorbed a future calendar that stretches five years down an uncertain road. The journey begins soon and I will start to count again… 60 months, 59, 58… 30, 29, 28… 3, 2, 1… Happy New Year 2009!

I cannot tell you how helpful and therapeutic it is for me to share these thoughts with friends and family. It lightens my load… I sincerely hope it does not inadvertently add to yours… In love and friendship… Bob."

Chapter 15

Did It Work?

As in the previous chapter, my earlier writings provide insight to the process and the personal thoughts as I moved into the post-chemotherapy stage.

I Digress One . . .

"Last Friday, Janie and I went to Houston for some poking, probing, bloodletting and picture-taking. Compared to our first visit, this was a piece of cake, lasting only a few hours from beginning to end. The purpose was to determine if, after surgery and 12 chemotherapy sessions, there were any critters lurking around. We went back on Monday to hear the results and guess what. . . . NO CRITTERS!!

Not only did my internal organs say 'cheese' for the camera, but everything looked precisely as it had before entering chemotherapy. Things like white cells, hemoglobin, platelets etc. had returned to normal and a 'tumor marker' that had been 2.5 before surgery is now zero.

Following our review with the cancer care team, my shirttail barely touched my backside as I scooted out the door and headed for the elevator. The nurse laughed and noted that I did not appear to be sticking around for any more fun and fellowship. Janie stayed behind for a few minutes to ask a couple of questions. When she inquired of the nurse as to my whereabouts, her response was 'Judging from the way he left here, he is probably already in the car'. She was not far wrong. I was extremely relieved and anxious to get on the road home and away from this wonderful, awful, miraculous, deadly place.

Ambivalent is not a word with enough strength to describe how I feel about the MD Anderson environment. One can sense the justifiable optimism and hope present in the staff, patients and families. Great strides are being made every single day in the search for cure and prevention. However, one can also see the human evidence of lives and families that are reaching the end of a slow and painful process. They have arrived in a place where hope is a distant memory and the future has shrunk to a matter of a few short years, or even months or weeks. There are too many young people in their teens and twenties going through the treatment maze with old duffers like me. There are too many good people (patients and loved ones) whose lives are being assaulted by this awful disease. One cannot escape the thought that virtually all of these people looked like me at some point... pink cheeks... good color... good energy... even free of the disease for varying periods of time.

I shared a dressing room with several patients in line for xrays. I spoke with one man for a couple of minutes. It was the 43rd day of this particular hospital stay. He had bone cancer. He had received a bone marrow transplant that failed. He had undergone two rounds of chemotherapy. He smiled and said he had lost his hair twice. He seemed alone, but we are all alone when going through the process. That is, except for a son and his father who were there that same day.

The son was probably mid-to-late forties. One could sense the loving concern he felt for his father as he assisted him in putting on his gown. The father's eyes were vacant and tired, no doubt indicating a continuing and lengthy battle with the disease. But, there they were... looking for answers at MDA, the best of the best... never seeming to give in... always assuming there is one more step to take... one more test... one more treatment... hope for a cure.

Respect, dignity, strength, perseverance and limitless hope are all words that describe these wonderful people. They provide a near-overdose of humility as I contemplate my relatively painless sojourn and the wonderful report we have just received. I want to jump up and shout at the good news, but am unable to do so because of the lump in my throat and the mist in my eyes. Please hold up these good people in your thoughts and prayers... they sure could use the help... and thanks for doing that for me over these last months... Your Friend, Bob."

I Digress Two . . .

"Yesterday was my second follow-up visit to MDA since ending chemo in mid-September. You've already heard results of the first 'slice and dice' utilizing labs, xrays and scans. We did all that again yesterday, but also added my one-year colonoscopy. Thankfully I slept through the whole thing. The results will come tomorrow, but I still have a couple of things I wanted to share with you. You may have noticed over the years that I find all manner of environmental minutae that cannot pass without some kind of thought or inspection on my part. I'm not sure if that means I am easily distracted or hyper-curious. It could also mean that any tiny flash of light will shine in a dimly-lit room.

I have often mentioned the heart-rending nature of a day at MDA, where one is confronted with hundreds and hundreds of hopeful, but often very ill, cancer patients. In the midst of all this hope, optimism and sadness, there is often humor.

I was called into the CT-Scan ante room with two others to complete administrative paperwork prior to the procedure. One of the two was a little woman who could not have been more than 4'10" and must have been over 80 years of age. As cute as she was in her colorful jacket, she was no doubt a mere shadow of her younger, more attractive self (sounds familiar). As we sat next to each other waiting our turn, I looked down at the magazine open on her lap. With pen in hand, one page at a time, she was obviously making selections from the pages of a Victoria's Secret catalog. I could not help but smile softly and privately at this picture of hope, optimism and, quite possibly, delusion (but that's okay at MDA).

It reminded me of an old joke that the absolute pinnacle of optimism is a professional accordion player with a beeper.

My second mental note comes as a warning to all who passed the age of majority about four decades ago. As I was going through my normal shine, shower and shave in the wee hours before the test maze started, I noticed some scary person staring back at me from the hotel mirror. In addition to the crevices (one step up from wrinkles) and various and sundry droops and folds, this imposter looked like he had been 'rode hard and put up wet'. Surely there was no one in our family who could look like they had that many miles on 'em and still be vertical. But there he was, in all his aging, gravity-winnin', high-mileage glory, lookin' like something the cat brought home for dinner. And then it hit me... fluorescent lighting... the enemy of all who wish to keep their blemishes a secret and reality hidden comfortably in subdued, indirect lighting. I thankfully recalled that our master bath not only has incandescent light, but it is also connected to a dimmer switch that I keep turned very, very low. I'm learning to shave in the dark and have become adept at moving around the house with only indirect lighting and the faint glow of the TV. I look great! And I haven't told anyone that my cosmetics counter has moved from Macy's to the caulk, putty and paint department at Home Depot.

Finally, I must pilfer from Lily Tomlin (Janie and I saw her show at the Bass Hall in Fort Worth). Seems an aging friend (in her 90's) in a nursing home had a couple of complaints. One was that she wanted to complain about the food but most residents thought it was great. Thus, she couldn't get any traction on that issue. The other issue was that she and a gentleman resident had developed a relationship that they wished to take to the next level of intimacy (please don't make me be more specific). When they tried to close the door to get some privacy, the staff would not allow them to close the door... thus her frustration. A friend's advice went something like this... 'the next time you feel moved to be intimate, simply go ahead and do it with the door open. I assure you that after a couple of times, the staff will close the door... '.

Hit that dimmer switch on the way out... will you? Hope your New Year is starting off with mucho positive gusto and thanks for allowing me to share... Bob."

Chapter 16

An End… A Beginning

Another note to family and friends:

"There are no findings to suggest presence of metastatic disease"... magical, wonderful, uplifting, optimistic, hopeful words. It was the lead sentence in a report on the outcome of tests administered earlier in the week. Excuse me while I do a couple of cartwheels and a little "end zone shuffle" just to let everyone know there is good news at the Cull household! My doctor was impressed with my pink shirt... and my pink cheeks. He feels confident enough to wait six months for the next CT scan and two years for the next colonoscopy. All in all, I simply could not ask for more at this stage.

As I have said many times before, there may be nothing to make one feel more conflicted than receiving extremely good news in the presence of so many people (young and old) receiving not-so-good news. Images that will remain... an early teen slumped over in a wheel chair being pushed by his dad, obviously exhausted from a chemotherapy session... running into a friend from years ago whose wife was diagnosed only after cancer had spread to most major organs in her body... a 74-year-old man who had undergone six surgeries in 2004... a young woman with deep-set eyes and dark circles underneath waited until I opened my resting eyes to let me know that the chair in which I was waiting (uncomfortably) for the CT scan was actually a recliner. Each is a member of a community of cancer patients, bonded through their common illness. They are determined to persevere through all manner of physical and emotional trauma to what they hope will be an ultimate victory over this illness. They are friendly and open and spirited. As we go through our day, we exchange pleasantries and smiles with virtually every person. We do so because at MDA there are no strangers… only cancer friends who are sharing the most intimate and critical stage in their lives and the lives of their loved ones. It is important to speak, but more important to listen. It is important to note every small victory with encouragement and hope. It is important to smile, to laugh and to recall positive and humorous history from each life. These are the markers for living life constructively and hopefully, and provide a different reality (a diversion) from the one more current and stark.

Each trip to MDA is one slice of a journey. Each slice has its own personality and character. And, each slice carries with it some enlightenment or new information about the path we are on and where it is leading. We are open to this new information only gradually. We experience an "ahaism" only when we are able to place it in our emotional "dittybag" without hitting overload. One such revelation that I finally understood (accepted) into my reality is that I will always be a cancer patient. Removing your appendix removes appendicitis. Removing your tonsils cures tonsilitis. But, once cancer has been detected, one will always be a cancer patient. Every test result or any anomaly in labs, xrays, scans or any other analytical test will be viewed differently forever. Symptomology or changes in virtually any aspect of physical functioning is viewed with caution and suspicion.

Please don't misunderstand. I am not complaining. Rather, I am simply now willing to absorb that reality and adjust my game plan to include a bit more diligence and awareness relative to health matters. That is a good thing, a positive development that will allow me to be a more effective partner in my own well-being.

But, the most important thing is that I remain grateful for all the thoughts and prayers that have been sent our way by friends and family. Regardless of the outcome, there is always comfort in knowing folks are holding good thoughts for you. And, as always, I hope you will share those same thoughts and prayers with all my special friends at MDA. . . Your Friend Bob."

Chapter 17

First and Last: Be A Blood Donor and Other Advice

Let me recommend that anyone out there who is able should donate blood. It is a good thing to do for altruistic reasons. It helps a lot of people get through life-threatening moments and contributes to their recovery. It makes you feel good to walk out of the blood center to the sound of "thank you" from the staff. You are energized by simply knowing you have done a good, unselfish thing for a perfect stranger. But let's be selfish for a moment.

Having been a donor for many years, I had become one of the "56-day" people who received a card a week or so in advance of each date on which I was eligible. My blood was so rich in red cells that I often gave something called "double red" that multiplied its use while not demanding any more from my body.

I gave in early November, 2003. My next eligibility date was early January, 2004, and I showed up about mid-month. For those who may not know, blood centers provide five pieces of information about your health (temperature, hemoglobin, coagulation, blood pressure and cholesterol). The first four can affect your ability to donate blood, while the latter is more of a "thank you" gift for showing up.

It was that January visit when they informed me that my hemoglobin had dropped below the normal range. Since this had never occurred in my lifetime, I asked them to take it a second time. The result was the same. I was anemic. At that moment, I understood why a couple of family members had asked if I was feeling well because I seemed a little pale.

This prompted a meeting with my internist, who immediately ordered a colonoscopy. Sure enough, a large tumor was the source of internal blood loss. In fairly rapid-fire order, we got lined up with a surgeon who put us on the schedule only days after my unwelcome discovery.

You may recall that this is the exact point where I made the case for involving a healthy partner in managing the disease process. The "we" referenced above includes me and my wife. Your "disease manager" could be a relative, a close friend or even a paid clinical professional. The need for this person is even more imperative when the patient is a healthcare "klutz" (guess who?) who has never had anything much more serious than a dry, hacking cough as evidence of poor health. Managing the process will take tireless research, an inquisitive and persistent mind and the ability to coordinate complex schedules and services. Involving that "disease manager" may be the single most important element in arriving at a successful conclusion. I know there may be some situations where this is simply not possible, but every alternative should be exhausted before negotiating this maze alone.

A second suggestion at this point is that you might seek out a personal "guide" that you can either emulate or actually get to walk with you in your journey. Ideally, this would be someone close at hand… someone you have observed and admired relative to their ability to handle challenges similar to your own. In my case, this was an individual who has had to live with diabetes his entire life. We have been friends and colleagues for about a dozen years or so. I have observed his attitude and demeanor over the years as he faced the daily (almost hourly) challenges of monitoring, measuring and administering required of diabetes patients. I saw his happiness as he moved from injections to a high-technology pump that could provide a much greater degree of control with substantially less effort. He has escaped some of the serious side effects of this debilitating disease (e.g.

amputations), but has suffered others (e.g. open heart surgery, impaired vision, etc.). I marvel at his ability to maintain a positive countenance, laugh at my jokes and continue to grow and evolve in spite of his healthcare burden.

He is one of my heroes. You should have one too.

Chapter 18

A Father's Day Letter To My Children

This letter is part of my Father's day gift to you. My hope is that the information contained in the letter and the materials that surround it will convey the depth and breadth of my love and concern for you. I have always felt privileged to be your Dad and want you to know that your uniqueness as individuals and your special natures continue to be a source of joy for me.

We are all acutely aware that the newest member of our family is colon cancer (actually Mimi introduced this family member initially). Please don't take what follows the wrong way. But if I should die from colon cancer that has metastasized in some other location in my body, you have the right and I encourage you to be extremely angry with me. I say this because I alone will have stolen precious years from my life as a dad, as a husband, as a brother and brother-in-law, as an uncle and as a grandfather. I am mortified that I have placed myself in harm's way for reasons known only to God and broccoli. I have been stubborn. I have been stupid. I have failed to follow the advice of your mother. I have failed even to do what my internist told me to do several years ago. I have ignored the massive amount of information available that tells us when, where and how often to have a colonoscopy done, and who is at greatest risk for this disease. This did not need to happen, at least at this time and in this manner.

Let me say that I honestly do not expect to die from colon cancer. As you are aware, there are many factual and good reasons to be optimistic that my recovery will be complete, that there will be no recurrence over the coming three years or so and that I will reestablish normal life expectancy at the end. I feel good. There is no evidence of cancer at this time. The chemotherapy is going well as to side-effects and everything points to a successful outcome. I have purchased OU tickets for next fall and your Mother and I have renewed symphony tickets for next year. So I have no intention of going anywhere in the near future.

Let me wrap up this part by saying that if I should die of anything other than colon cancer or its metastasizing, remember me fondly and without anger. However, I will allow you to be a little ticked for having dragged you through a rather scary experience.

The second part of what I want to say deals more with you, your familial connection to the disease of colon cancer and what you must do to avoid the same kind of result. Your mother and I, your siblings, your spouses, your children and your friends care too much to let it slide as I have done. YOU MUST NOT ALLOW THAT TO HAPPEN! AND YOU MUST ENCOURAGE AND CAJOLE ONE ANOTHER IN A LOVING WAY TO STICK TO A PLAN.

Included here is a substantial amount of information about colon cancer and the examinations that are involved with diagnosis. It tells you when you should start and how often you should have the examinations. There are several procedures available. But let me say that a colonoscopy is head and shoulders above anything else for being certain to catch anything before it becomes cancerous and life threatening. That may change in the future, but do extensive research before accepting any other procedure.

My Father's Day wish is that you will seriously review the information, speak with a physician about your family history and develop a plan for when you will have your first colonoscopy. If you do not do this, then I have the right to be angry. You now know more about the disease than most. You know it is virtually 100% preventable if you follow a strict regimen of examination. There is really no reason to die from this disease.

Is it possible to end something like this with "Happy Father's Day"? I believe maybe more than ever. Hopefully, my optimism about beating this thing will be justified and you will be sensitized in a way that may not have been possible otherwise. That would indeed be a "happy" result . . .

Chapter 19

One More Thing… Maybe Two

As I neared that moment when the manuscript would suddenly become "final", I realized that there were a number of items that had not found a home in the text to this point. None of them are more or less important than any other, but they do represent some of the most current developments and communications around my status. Following one of my six-month "slice and dice" visits to MD Anderson, I imposed the following message on my Sunday School class:

> *"As many of you know, I went to MD Anderson on Monday for six-month tests, and returned on Wednesday to meet with the doctor and get the results. Thus, my email is divided into "test day" and "results day".*

Wednesday, 1/25: Boredom Is Good

In a time of fast-paced lifestyles and a constant search for creative innovations to satisfy our every whim, a little boredom can be a very good thing. I was in Houston Wednesday. I got a boring report from the doctor that said everything was exactly as it had been the last time… and the time before. It is about the only facet of my life in which I am seeking complete and utter boredom… absolutely nothing new to discuss… we'll see you in six months… have a safe trip. A deep sigh of relief left me feeling a bit exhausted as it always does during the few days around my tests and their results. As accomplished as I may be at pushing my mind over, under, around and through scary stuff, there is an emotional tension just under the surface that drains the tank a bit.

Tuesday, 1/24: Thenk You Vuurry Much

Like Elvis says it (present tense… he's alive you know). I got a nice birthday postcard from the class VP of happy stuff… there was a great big "37" printed in the upper right corner. Thought to myself (as I hit the flex pose and strutted in front of the mirror) "man, do I have 'em fooled… but I do look pretty dadgum good". Then Janie explained that was just how they printed the postage on postcards. She also explained that she had put up a poster of Troy Aikman in place of the mirror. Reality again… who needs it.

I just returned from one day of blood, scan and xray testing fun at MD Anderson in Houston… regular six month evaluation. As per usual, I return on Wednesday to meet with the doc and discuss the results. I've decided (a la Letterman) that my top ten worst words are on the CT scan table... "lower your pants and turn over on your left side". What follows is the placement of a slender, cold device where the sun don't shine. This is administered by a perfect stranger who has no business whatsoever seein' what she's seein' or doin' what she's doin'. I could swear I heard a muffled giggle... or maybe it was a cackle.

The scan is always the last test on the schedule. It takes me about 1 minute, 32.7 seconds to cover the half-mile of skybridges and hallways that get me back to the hotel, the parking garage and on the freeway back to Mansfield. I would take one of those inside shuttle things but they don't move fast enough. I nearly burn up a pair of deck shoes on each trip (that's right, deck shoes... I keep a pair just in case I ever have a boat deck to stand on). Ok, so I have an ascot and a smoking jacket too... just in case I wanta smoke and look reeeallllly good at the same time.

While I was waiting for the little witc... er, angel... to draw blood, I was on one of those recliners staring up at the ceiling. I noticed a message in big, bold letters attached to a plastic covering over the two light fixtures.

The message said "Contractor: This plastic sheeting is to protect the louvers during installation… please remove before turning on the light fixture". It was real easy to read because the light was on behind the plastic wrapping. Soooo, I have nothing new to report on the contracting business.

I went through the same drill as always on the barium … nurse says "Which flavor do you want?"… I say "What are the flavors?"… nurse says "banana, berry, apple and the original"… I say "What's the 'original' "?… she says, "orange"… I say "Give me the original". I can never remember the flavors for six months and can't figure out why they can't just say "orange" in the first place.

I guess it's becoming apparent that I'm easily entertained. As always, I also came away inspired by a stranger. As I waited to see my doctor, an older gentleman (must have been at least a year or two older than me) came through the door. He was thin, frail and pale but he had a big smile on his face. A younger man waited for him with a wheel chair. He proclaimed loudly to his companion, "Man! I can't tell you how happy and relieved I am that they are going to do it!!!" He repeated similar words several times as he was wheeled off toward the elevators. He was obviously very ill, but was just as obviously thrilled that they were going to do "it". I do not know what "it" is. But, if I were going to guess, given his appearance and diminished health status, I would speculate that "it" is probably some kind of surgery or a fairly serious chemotherapy regimen. And he was thrilled… not just pleased… THRILLED!!!!! Once again, I was reminded by a fellow traveler to make one more big deposit in my "grateful" account. I am so very grateful for my continued good fortune in dealing with my own circumstance. But I am also grateful for having been sitting outside that door when that courageous and spirited soulmate announced to all within earshot that his spirit was alive and well inside that diminished physical body. It is a life lesson for all of us… Be well…"

I suppose what follows could be the "… Maybe Two" part of the chapter title. While it is still on the subject, it also speaks to the need for us to surround ourselves with "soul food". It kind of went like this:

"I had a friend who once said of me "when you leave the room, those remaining know they have bought something... they may not be quite sure what it is but they know they've bought it". I always considered that the highest compliment anyone has ever given me because it speaks not only of skill, but credibility, believability and sincerity.

I have spent the last couple of days trying to figure out exactly what I "bought" on Sunday. The tandem of Don's nudge to discover our "soul food" followed by Meg's stirring, insightful and humorous description of her battle with cancer was almost overwhelming to the senses... at least my senses.

Don very effectively took what could be a complex topic and found a way to delineate and define the soul in language even I could understand. Those things that put a lump in your throat, a tear in your eye, a smile on your face, joy in your heart (mind) or a bounce in your step all qualify as "soul food". I have been thinking since then about those items that are on my "soul food" menu, and I wanted to share one of those.

Little children, with our four grandchildren being first among equals, are the stuff of "soul food" for me.

When I am in the presence of small children, the rest of the world literally goes away. The day's headlines, man's inhumanity to man and any personal challenges currently on the agenda simply go up in a puff of smoke when little children are present. Those things really don't disappear. Rather they are swallowed up in the glow of unconditional love, infinite curiosity, boundless energy, amazing creativity and a continuing celebration of time and space defined as this moment and no other... completely free from both the past and the future. Their eyes are bright, their smiles are bountiful, their giggles are infectious and their hugs envelop your soul when their little arms cannot reach around you physically.

Thank you, Don, for prompting me to think a bit differently about "soul food" and what that means to the way I live my life.

Listening to Meg's story is another form of "soul food". It was inspiring and hopeful and optimistic. She had some really funny lines interspersed with a more serious message. But I had difficulty laughing because I wanted to cry. I spent almost the entire time swallowing hard to maintain my composure, hoping not to break out in a full "blubber" and detract from her outstanding message. It is unclear to me why I reacted the way I did. After some thought, I believe it may be that her story brought a rush of memories. The memories were not so much of my own journey, which is pale by comparison. Rather it was the memory of those hundreds and thousands of cancer patients, many of whom are not alive to tell their story today. She is a young person, and it brought back memories of the many young people struggling with this killer far too early in their lives.

But she is here and I am here due to the six elements she identified as necessary for survival. I believe they were doctors, technology, medicine, faith, love and luck. My soul was fed by her story, which will be uplifting to all who hear it.

I hope you all don't mind my taking a few moments of your time to share my thoughts... it simply seemed like Sunday was a big day for me... your friend Bob."

Chapter 20

When Only Words Remain

It is not my intent to end the book in a way that detracts from the optimism, hope and humor that pushes me to live life productively and constructively. But it occurred to me that not all stories end in the same place… nor do they all have a result that can be easily accepted or understood by those left behind. That recognition created an urge to share some of my very personal and private communications to others who had lost friends and loved ones during this time of challenge. Of course, the names will change to protect their privacy. I do not know that this will be helpful in any way. But my thought is that those who are in desperate circumstances or who have been left behind when a loved one is lost may find some "nugget" that will help them to rebuild their spirit. Short of that, it may simply help to know that the emotional roller coaster on which you find yourself is one that many of us have traveled. You are not alone. What follows is a series of writings, some to an individual and others to a larger group.

> *"I want to tell you that Harry can't dance. He has danced through our lives for so long with such grace and graciousness that it is difficult to accept. Earlier this week, he suffered a loss of equilibrium brought on by cancer that*

has traveled to a place that affects his balance. Our dear friend needs us physically and prayerfully. He has taken up residence in Room 3222 at Arlington Memorial Hospital to continue the battle with an aggressive and unrelenting cancer. Although not feeling up to par, he has put out the "Visitor's Welcome" mat and would enjoy seeing folks for a few minutes if you get the chance.

It is important that we continue to lift Harry up in our thoughts and prayers as we go through the days ahead. We all want many more encores from this deeply spiritual man who has always danced the dance of his faithful professions. Beyond that, we want Harry to feel the warmth and peace of our unflinching admiration, love and respect for one who has so gracefully waltzed with us for so many years. . . . Your friend, Bob."

Another to my Aldersgate friends:

"Joyce. Duane. Mr. Bresden. Harry. We were hundreds of miles away geographically. But we were as close as close can be in our hearts. You all knew Joyce and Harry. You didn't know Duane or Mr. Bresden, the former a decades long friend and the latter a 97-year-old icon/father of a decades long friend. I want to say "stop"... "wait just a minute"… "please give us just a little time to catch our emotional breath". All this has occurred in a few short weeks. It moves too quickly. It challenges our faith and our ability to find peace in constant and irrevocable loss. But find peace we must… move on carrying the spirit of those departed we must… believe that footprints left will guide our future we must… rediscover gratefulness for life itself we must… rediscover loved ones remaining we must.

Finally, it occurs to me that we also <u>should.</u> It is the will of those who are no longer here. It is the example of those as well. If we were unable to achieve all that and more, those spirits would be saddened by our lack of understanding and will. They are indeed special souls, each in its own right, each in its own way. While small in stature, Harry fills the "suit of soul" to its limits and beyond. He was special to our class as a friend and as a near perfect example of what it means to be Christian. Soft-spoken and unassuming, he was nevertheless a significant presence in each of our spiritual lives. More than that, he was significant in the life of our church. He was special indeed.

I am taking the liberty of ending with an email sent to the long-time friend whose father died. You will note that I speak of his generation, which is the same as my Dad. While I recognize that neither Harry nor Joyce were in the same age group (although Harry was closer), the things I said apply equally. It is my belief that every generation has those who cast "long shadows" and who leave the world a better place for their having been here. I believe Harry and Joyce are among those.

"A Gathering of Long Shadows

Dear Friend:

I can never think of your Dad without thinking of my own. Both men totally committed to their families. Both totally committed to the communities they served. Both leaders politically and spiritually. Both absolutely and completely immersed in their chosen profession. Remarkable men in a remarkable generation. My Dad lived barely over half as long as your own. Both cast a very long shadow… living out their exemplary and successful lives while maintaining the highest levels of professionalism, integrity, character and ethics. But maybe the most striking characteristic of all was their humility. They expected no less of themselves and felt a sense of responsibility for their communities and their country. While certainly enjoying their success on some levels, their true joy was derived from the contribution they were able to make to those around them. In many ways, they were servants of the greater good, often giving more of themselves than anyone had a right to expect... but always joyful in their giving.

Our Dads were accompanied on their journey by other strong men and women of that unique generation. Their contribution cannot be diminished or underestimated. In the end, however, the ultimate generational achievements, as in any endeavor, must be led by the few. Our Dads were among the few, stepping out from every crowd, moving forward with optimism and hope and encouraging those around them to share in the effort and in the achievement. Remarkable men indeed.

Somewhere beyond our comprehension there is a place where long shadows gather. I feel in my heart that your Dad and mine are among those who cast them, along with other special souls who have gone this way. We will all miss your Dad, but feel fortunate to have known and experienced his presence and his friendship for so many wonderful years. Your friend... Bob."

I know that each of you reading this knows of someone who casts a long shadow. Whether they are still with us or have gone to a place they have earned through their words and deeds, their long shadows still provide markers to guide our aspirations.

EPILOGUE AND MY EPIPHANY

If you have pulled yourself through my treatise (some might say "knothole"), you have both my appreciation and the hope that you feel the trip was worthwhile. If you liked what you saw, I will take the credit. If not, you can blame the friends and family who encouraged me to share my writings with a broader audience.

I am ambivalent about this work even as I reach the end of it. The ambivalence stems from the fact that I am one of the truly fortunate cancer patients who have gone through the early stages of diagnosis, surgery and chemotherapy with minimal suffering and a prognosis that looks reassuring. At the moment the test results, scans and other data are absent any indications that the disease is still hanging around and there is no reason to believe that will change.

On the other hand, there are no guarantees once you have embarked on this journey. Each of us has chosen a method of dealing with our circumstance. By reading this, you have seen mine. If by sharing the view from my "window" I can provide a couple of "aha's" and a chuckle or two, it is worth the effort. If you find a helpful hint or become more aware that you are not alone, it is worth the effort. As I mentioned earlier, simply expressing my feelings and experiences in writing helps to lighten my load. I sincerely hope that reading this book has helped to lighten yours. Finally, I shared the following epiphany with friends:

"Every six months for the next few years, I will travel to MDA for labs, scans and x-rays to closely monitor any changes in my condition. I did that this week and can thankfully report that there is nothing new to report. I got to read those wonderful words . . "No evidence of metastatic or recurrent disease" one more time.

You know that I struggle with the idea that things are going so well for me when people like Harry, Allen, Horace, Janeen and hundreds of MDA patients I see on each visit are struggling with complications and challenges that would scuttle most of us. I am thrilled to hear the words quoted above but feel ambivalent given the knowledge that others are not so fortunate at the moment.

I am a slow learner (Janie could have told you that a long time ago), so only now have I come to realize something that is both real and liberating. In the simplest terms, it is "my happiness is your happiness".

As I dutifully choked down my three cups of barium, I was in the presence of two patients. One is suffering with the after-effects of removing part of her stomach and part of her esophagus. The other is a colon cancer patient like me. The former was told two years ago that she had two weeks to live.

Both were cheerful and communicative. We saw numerous patients come and go, many of whom were in very serious condition. As we each described our journey, it was obvious that they were very happy to hear that things had been going well for me. A third patient in the xray waiting area was a 26-year-old young woman who had been coming to MDA for years. All the technicians knew her first name and greeted her with a big hug. With a bright smile and a joyful countenance, she recalled a time when, as a little girl, her file was so thick that she had difficulty carrying it from one testing area to the next. MDA is now paperless, and all she carries is a Bible. I had never met those patients before, but they knew me. We may never meet again but we will never forget each other. We don't know each other's names but we will never forget the face or the story that came with it. But, most importantly, they were truly happy for me and clearly would hold me up in their prayers and thoughts for continuing good news in the future. I will do the same for them.

My epiphany came in looking back at those moments. My good fortune does not discourage those in more difficult circumstances. It does not create envy or antagonism. Rather, it creates joy and hope. They become a part of your celebration of life. Rather than retreat into frustration or sadness, they join your party and drink Margaritas and dance all night.

Each one of us who is on this journey is connected in the spirit in ways that escape my understanding, but is nevertheless real. We don't know each other, but we KNOW each other. 'My Happiness Is Your Happiness'... 'Your Happiness Is My Happiness'. That is one thing friends and fellow travelers share at the very center of our being."

Godspeed to you, your loved ones and your caregivers as you go forward with resolve and abundant hope... Your fellow traveler... Bob Cull."

ACKNOWLEDGEMENTS

Asking forgiveness from those I may leave out, let me offer my sincere and heartfelt appreciation to a number of important people in my life and in this endeavor.

First, I must pay tribute to Janie, my wife of 41 years, who combined a caring heart and a strong sense of nurturing with healthcare knowledge and a stubborn, results-oriented focus. She helped drive the entire process from diagnosis to treatment and beyond. One would be hard-pressed to convince me that our experience would have had the same positive outcome without her presence.

Still first among equals are my children, who frequently offered their assistance and continuously provided encouragement and optimism to bolster my spirit. They cheered me on in all the right places and in all the right ways. Beyond that, my children and grandchildren provided me the strength and dedication to step through this challenge simply by their existence. They are not special because they are perfect. They are special because they are mine. My life would not be pointless without them, but would, in my view, be diminished.

My sister and her family, along with extended family members all provided support. Added to that is what I consider to be "family" by extension. Members of our Aldersgate Sunday School class of many years at Trinity United Methodist Church in Arlington, Texas, stood with us throughout, offering food, prayers and positive thoughts along the way. They also tolerated my email musings, laughing and crying with me as I shared this experience.

I cannot stop without acknowledging the wonderful caregivers who all played a role in doing the things necessary to fend off and defeat this disease. Physicians, nurses and technicians with many different skills extended themselves at every turn to make an unpleasant journey as pleasant as possible. Most importantly, they were intensely focused on restoring my good health and returning me to many more years of life on the planet.

Finally, I must thank the hundreds of fellow travelers at MD Anderson and UT Southwestern who helped me to see that, regardless of circumstances, there is always hope, optimism and purpose in our being.

Thanks to you all.

ABOUT THE AUTHOR

Robert E. "Bob" Cull was born and raised in Frederick, Oklahoma, a small southwestern Oklahoma community. The second child born into a daily newspaper family, his exposure to words, language and written expression was an integral part of his environment during those early years.

As a young adult, he was called on to manage the same newspaper that his father had managed before him, providing additional opportunities to hone his writing skills. Subsequent choices led him away from that small community and into the larger world of work in Denver, Colorado. He ultimately enrolled at the University of Colorado, earning both a BS and MBA from that institution.

His professional path has involved a fair amount of marketing and business-to-business sales in the early years, evolving into executive roles in marketing and operations in the healthcare field. Still fully engaged running a small company, his hope is to return to his roots. His goal is to create a volume of written work covering a wide range of topics that can be helpful, informative, inspirational or provocative.

You can visit his web site at *www.bobcull.com* to sample his written work and find out about his latest offerings.

WHAT OTHERS ARE SAYING

"I just wanted you to know how much I enjoyed your manuscript about colon cancer. I wanted to let you know how insightful I thought it was and how I really believe your words will be able to help so many people get through the whole ordeal."

And another... "I just finished your book. I'm on my way out the door but I wanted to send you a note to say I LOVED IT!! I think there is much promise here and I feel very privileged to have gotten to read it... It is funny, thought-provoking, funny, educational, and did I say funny???"

"Just reading the Table of Contents is enough to make me buy the book. I just have to know what in the world is driving those Chapter titles."

"... you are the most gifted writer to spring forth with such a sensitive and beautiful message... "

WEBSITES

Mark Elliott Miller, fellow author ("The Husband's Guide to Cancer Survival"), had compiled a list of internet sites that are particularly useful to cancer patients, loved ones and caregivers as they work their way through the complex challenges of this disease. I repeat them here, and hope you will find them useful in your search for information and understanding.

American Assn. For Marriage & Family Therapists

www.aamft.org

American Cancer Society

www.cancer.org

Hospice Foundation of America

www.hospicefoundation.org

International Myeloma Foundation

www.myeloma.org

Susan B. Komen Breast Cancer Foundation

www.komen.org

Leukemia & Lymphoma Society

www.leukemia.org

Mayo Clinic

www.mayoclinic.com

MD Anderson Cancer Center

www.mdanderson.org

Memorial Sloan-Kettering Cancer Center

www.mskcc.org

Multiple Myeloma Research Foundation

www.multiplemyeloma.org

National Association of Social Workers

www.socialworkers.org

National Cancer Institute

www.cancer.gov

National Center for Grieving Children & Families

www.grievingchild.org

National Cervical Cancer Coalition

www.nccc-online.org

National Hospice & Palliative Care Organization

www.nhpco.org

National Ovarian Cancer Coalition

www.ovarian.org

Society of Gynecologic Oncologists

www.sgo.org

United Way of America

www.national.unitedway.org/myuw